The Ultimate Dash Diet Cookbook

Simple and Quick Recipes to enjoy your Dash Diet Plan

Natalie Puckett

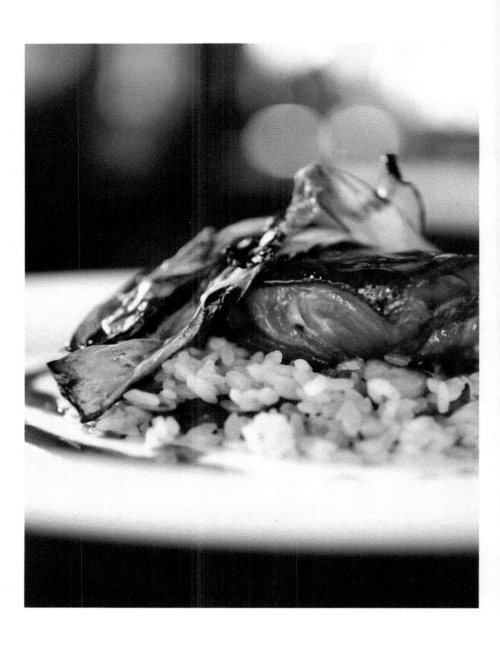

Table of Contents

Grilled Miso-Glazed Cod

SmartPoints value: Green plan - 3SP, Blue plan - 2SP, Purple plan - 2SP

Total Time: 35 min, Prep time: 10 min, Cooking time: 15 min, Serves: 4

Nutritional value: Cal - 227.2, Carbs - 15.0g, Fat - 3.1g, Protein - 30.0g

Ingredients

White miso - 3 Tbsp

Sugar (dark brown) - 1½ Tbsp

Sake - 1 Tbsp

Mirin - ½ fl oz, (1 Tbsp)

Atlantic cod (uncooked) - 20 oz, (fillets, skin removed

Cooking spray - 1 spray(s)

Uncooked scallion(s) (chopped) - 2 Tbsp

Instructions

1.   Whisk together miso, sugar, sake, and mirin in a small bowl and spread the mixture over the cod. Cover the cod and refrigerate for at least 2 hours or up to 24 hours.

2.   Coat a grill pan off the heat with cooking spray and preheat to medium heat.

3.   Remove the cod from marinade (reserve marinade). Place it in a fish grilling basket and grill until the cod is opaque and flakes easily with a fork.

4.   Grill each side for about 5 to 7 min (brush the cod with the remaining marinade half-way through the grilling phase to create a thicker glaze). Serve the cod garnished with scallions.

Grilled Tuna with Herb Butter

SmartPoints value: Green plan - 4SP, Blue plan - 3SP, Purple plan - 3SP

Total Time: 18 min, Prep time: 12 min, Cooking time: 6 min, Serves: 4

Nutritional value: Calories - 192.0, Carbs - 8.3g, Fat - 2.5g, Protein - 38.3g

Ingredients

Olive oil - 1 tsp

Lime juice (fresh) - 1 tsp

Black pepper - ⅛ tsp, or to taste

Cooking spray - 1 spray(s)

Salted butter - 2 Tbsp, softened

Chives (finely chopped) - 1 Tbsp, fresh

Parsley (fresh) - 1 Tbsp, finely chopped

Tarragon (fresh) - 1 Tbsp, finely chopped

Lime zest (fresh, minced) - 1 tsp

Table salt - ¼ tsp, or to taste

Spinach (fresh) - 1 pound(s), baby-variety, steamed

Yellowfin tuna (uncooked) - 1 pound(s), one steak cut 1- to 1-1/2 inches thick

Instructions

1.   Drizzle oil and lime juice on both sides of the fish and set it aside.

2.   Coat your grill with cooking spray off heat, and preheat the grill on high heat.

3.   Combine softened butter, chives, parsley, tarragon, lime zest, salt, and pepper in a small metal bowl and then set aside.

4.   Grill the tuna on one side for three minutes, then carefully turn it and cook on the other side for another three minutes or longer until you have achieved the desired degree of cooking.

5.   Place the bowl containing butter mixture on the grill just until it melts. Don't let it cook.

6.   Slice the tuna thinly and serve it over spinach, then drizzle melted herb butter over the top.

Lemon-Herb Roasted Salmon

SmartPoints value: Green plan - 5SP, Blue plan - 2SP, Purple plan - 2SP

Total Time: 31 min, Prep time: 16 min, Cooking time: 15 min, Serves: 4

Nutritional value: Calories - 118.1, Carbs - 1.0g, Fat - 6.8g, Protein - 12.9g

Ingredients

Black pepper (coarsely ground) - ⅛ tsp (or to taste)

Cooking spray - 1 spray(s)

Lemon juice (fresh) - 4 Tbsp, divided

Lemon zest (finely grated) - 1 tsp (with extra for garnish, if you like)

Minced garlic - 1 tsp

Oregano (fresh) - 1 tsp

Parsley (fresh, chopped) - 1 Tbsp (with extra for garnish, if you like)

Uncooked wild pink salmon fillet(s) (also known as humpback salmon) - 1½ pound(s), four 6-oz pieces about 1-inch-thick each

Table salt - ⅛ tsp (or to taste)

Sugar - 1½ Tbsp

Thyme (fresh, chopped) - 1 Tbsp (with extra for garnish, if you like)

Instructions

1.   Heat your oven to 400°F before using it. Get a small, shallow baking dish and coat it with cooking spray.

2.   Apply seasoning to both sides of the salmon with salt and pepper, then place the salmon in the prepared baking dish and drizzle on it with two tablespoons of lemon juice.

3.   Whisk the remaining two tablespoons of lemon juice, sugar, parsley, thyme, lemon zest, garlic, and oregano together in a small bowl, then continue whisking until the sugar dissolves in the mixture and set it aside.

4.   Roast the salmon until it is close to being ready; about 13 minutes, then remove it from the oven and top it with the lemon-herb mixture.

5.   Return it to the oven and allow it to roast until the salmon is fork-tender, about 2 minutes more. Garnish the dish with fresh herbs that you chopped and the grated zest, if you like.

Grilled Tuna Provencal

SmartPoints value: Green plan - 3SP, Blue plan - 2SP, Purple plan - 2SP

Total Time: 20 min, Prep time: 10 min, Cooking time: 10 min, Serves: 4

Nutritional value: Calories - 335, Carbs - 14.6g, Fat - 15.5g, Protein - 36.1g

Ingredients

Black pepper (freshly ground, divided) - ¾ tsp

Cooking spray - 3 spray(s)

Uncooked tuna (about 1- to 1 1/2-in thick) - 1 pound(s)

Olive(s) (pitted and chopped)- 6 large

Olive oil - 1 Tbsp

Rosemary (fresh, minced) - 1 Tbsp

Red wine - 2 fl oz

Sea salt - ¾ tsp, divided

Tomato(es) (fresh, diced) - 2½ cup(s)

Garlic clove(s) (minced) - 2 medium clove(s)

Parsley (fresh, minced) - 2 Tbsp

Sugar - ⅛ tsp

Instructions

1.　　Wash the tuna thoroughly and pat it dry. Rub 1/4 teaspoon each of salt and pepper over it, then set it aside.

2.　　Combine tomatoes, parsley, rosemary, garlic, olives, oil, and the remaining 1/2 teaspoon each of salt and pepper in a separate bowl, then set it aside.

3.　　Get a reasonably large grill pan and coat it with cooking spray, then set it over medium-high heat. When the pan is visibly hot, cook the tuna for 2 to 3 minutes (or longer) per side for a rare cook (or thorough cook). As soon as you have prepared the tuna, remove it to a serving plate and wrap it with aluminum foil to keep it warm.

4.　　Add the red wine, tomato mixture, and sugar to the hot grill pan and cook, scraping the bottom of the pan frequently, until the tomato mixture reduces to about two cups. The alcohol must have cooked off.

5.　　Remove foil from the tuna, slice it thinly, and serve with tomato mixture over the top.

Southern-Style Oven-Fried Chicken

SmartPoints value: Green plan - 4SP, Blue Plan - 3SP, Purple plan - 3SP

Total Time: 45 min, Prep time: 15 min, Cooking time: 30 min, Serves: 4

Nutritional value: Calories - 256.9, Carbs - 31.3g, Fat - 1.6g, Protein - 27.5g

Switch to oven frying and lighten up this favorite hearty dish. I decided to improve the flavor by adding buttermilk and a pinch of cayenne pepper.

Ingredients

All-purpose flour - ⅓ cup(s)

Buttermilk (low-fat) - 3 oz

Cayenne pepper - ¼ tsp (or to taste), divided

Cooking spray - 3 spray(s)

Cornflake crumbs - ½ cup(s)

Table salt - ½ tsp (or to taste), divided

Uncooked chicken breast(s) - 1 pound(s), four 4-oz pieces (boneless, skinless)

Instructions

1.   Heat the oven to 375°F before starting. Coat a 13- X 8- X 2-inch baking dish lightly with cooking spray and set it aside.

2.   Add salt and cayenne pepper to chicken for a tasty seasoning and set it aside also.

3.   Put a mixture of flour, 1/4 teaspoon salt, and 1/8 teaspoon cayenne pepper in a bowl of medium size.

4.   Put the buttermilk and cornflakes crumbs in 2 separate shallow bowls.

5.   Dip the chicken in the flour mixture and evenly coat both sides.

6.   Next, dip the flour-coated chicken into buttermilk and turn it to coat both sides.

7.   Finally, dip the coated chicken in cornflake crumbs and turn to coat both sides.

8.   Place coated chicken breasts in the baking dish that you prepared.

9.   Bake the chicken until it is tender and no longer pink in the center (you don't need to flip the chicken while baking). The baking should take about 25 to 30 minutes.

Italian Chicken Soup with Vegetables

SmartPoints value: Green plan - 4SP, Blue plan - 1SP, Purple plan - 1SP

Total Time: 27 min, Prep time: 15 min, Cooking time: 12 min, Serves: 1

Nutritional value: Calories - 136.7, Carbs - 22.3g, Fat - 1.0g, Protein - 9.6g

Ingredients

Chicken broth - 1 cup(s), canned

Chicken breast(s) - 1 cup(s), diced (skinless, boneless)

Extra virgin olive oil - 1 tsp, divided

Fresh thyme - 1¼ tsp (leaves)

Fresh mushroom(s) - 1 cup(s), sliced

Garlic clove(s) - 1 medium-sized, minced

Green beans - 1 small bowl, cooked

Lemon(s) - 1 slice(s)

Plum tomato(es) - 1 medium-sized, diced

Uncooked cauliflower - 1 cup(s), small florets

Instructions

1.   Heat 1/2 tsp of olive oil in a small skillet over medium heat.

2.   Add the mushrooms and garlic, then cook, continuously stirring until mushrooms begin to soften and the mixture is fragrant; about 2 minutes.

3.   Add the broth in the chicken and bring it to a boil over medium-high heat.

4.   Add cauliflower and (or) green beans, then reduce the heat to medium-low and simmer until it is almost tender; about 4 minutes.

5.   Add the chicken, thyme, and tomatoes, then simmer until the vegetables are tender; about 2 minutes.

6.   Drizzle it with the remaining 1/2 tsp of oil and fresh lemon juice, then grind the pepper over the top, if you desire.

Roasted Chicken Breast with Spiced Cauliflower

SmartPoints value: Green plan - 4SP, Blue plan - 2SP, Purple plan - 2SP

Total Time: 50 min, Prep time: 20 min, Cooking time: 30 min, Serves: 4

Nutritional value: Calories - 470.9, Carbs - 3.5g, Fat - 11.3g, Protein - 84.2g

Ingredients

Black pepper (divided) - ½ tsp

Cayenne pepper - ⅛ tsp

Cooking spray - 2 spray(s)

Cilantro (finely chopped) - 1 Tbsp

Olive oil - 2 Tbsp

Coriander (ground) - 1 tsp

Turmeric (ground) - 1 tsp

Durkee Cumin (ground) - ½ tsp

Kosher salt (divided) - ¾ tsp

Uncooked chicken breast - 1 pound(s), two 8 oz pieces (boneless, skinless)

Uncooked cauliflower - 1 pound(s), cut into bite-size pieces

Fresh lime(s) - ½ medium, with wedges for serving

Instructions

1.   Before you start, heat the oven to 450°F. Get a large baking sheet and line it with parchment paper.

2.   Combine and mix oil, turmeric, coriander, cumin, 1/2 tsp of salt, 1/4 tsp of pepper, and cayenne in a large bowl.

3.   Place the chicken in the center of the prepared baking sheet and brush each piece with 1/2 tsp of oil mixture.

4.   Add cauliflower to the bowl and toss it to coat. Place the cauliflower around the chicken and lightly coat both chicken and cauliflower with cooking spray.

5.   Sprinkle the chicken with the remaining 1/4 tsp of each salt and pepper.

6.   Roast the coated chicken until it cooks through; 15-20 minutes and let it rest.

7.   Toss the cauliflower and chicken juices in the pan, then continue roasting until browned and tender; about 10 minutes more.

8.   Add the cilantro and toss again.

9.   Thickly slice the chicken across the grain and fan over

serving plates.

10. Serve the cauliflower and chicken in each plate and squeeze 1/2 lime over the top, then serve with additional lime wedges.

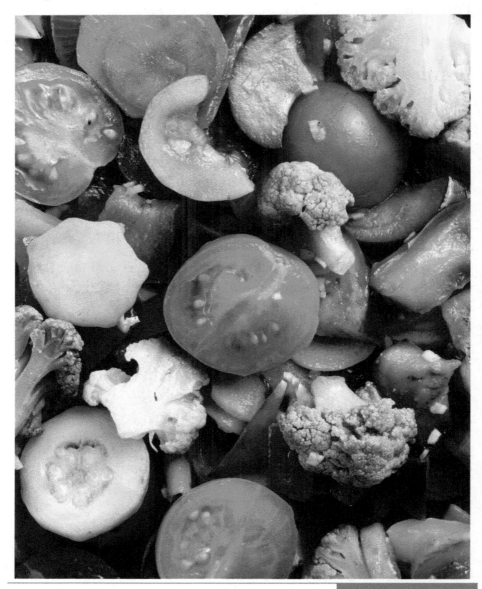

Vietnamese Chicken and Veggie Bowl with Rice Noodles

SmartPoints value: Green plan - 6SP, Blue plan - 4SP, Purple plan - 4SP

Total Time: 26 min, Prep time: 20 min, Cooking time: 6 min, Serves: 1

Nutritional value: Calories - 280.4, Carbs - 42.3g, Fat - 10.0g, Protein - 9.1g

Ingredients

Cilantro (chopped, fresh leaves) - 2 Tbsp

Cooked rice noodles - ½ cup(s)

Asian fish sauce - ½ tsp

Cooking spray - 4 spray(s)

Uncooked chicken breast - 5 oz, thin cutlet (boneless, skinless)

Uncooked broccoli - 1 cup(s), small florets or baby stalks

Red pepper(s) (sweet) - ½ medium, cut in 2 even pieces

Soy sauce (low sodium) - 2 Tbsp, divided (or to taste)

Sriracha sauce - 1 tsp (or to taste)

Sugar - ¼ tsp

Roasted peanuts (unsalted dry) - 2 tsp, chopped

Instructions

1.   Coat a grill or grill pan with cooking spray and preheat on medium-high heat.

2.   Place the chicken, broccoli, and red pepper in a shallow bowl and drizzle with one tablespoon of soy sauce, then toss to coat.

3.   Coat the chicken with cooking spray and grill, turning the chicken once and the vegetables a few times, until chicken cooks through and veggies are tender-crisp; about 6 minutes.

4.   Slice the chicken and pepper them into strips, then place all in a bowl over noodles.

5.   Stir together the remaining one tablespoon of soy sauce, fish sauce, and sugar. Drizzle the mixture over your cooked chicken.

Sprinkle a mixture of cilantro, peanuts, and sriracha on the chicken, then serve.

Fall Harvest Salad

SmartPoints value: Green plan - 3SP, Blue plan - 1SP, Purple plan - 1SP

Total time: 15 min, Prep time: 15 min, Cooking time: 0 min, Serves: 4

Nutritional value: Calories - 175, Carbs – 25.7g, Fat – 7.6g, Protein – 4.8g

Ingredients

Kale greens (baby variety) - 4-5 cups

Large apple (thinly sliced) - 1 piece

Sweet pumpkin seeds (toasted) - 1/3 cup

For dressing

Olive oil - 1 tbsp

Maple Syrup - 1 tbsp

Red wine vinegar - 2 tbsp

Shallot (minced) - 1 piece

Cinnamon - ¼ tsp

Dijon mustard - 1 tsp

Pepper and salt to taste

Instructions

1.   Beat all the ingredients for the dressing together in a small bowl

2.   Toss the ingredients for the salad in a large bowl

3.   Pour the processed dressing over the salad and toss to coat evenly

4.   This perfect dish is sure to impress your guests and compliment your holiday meal. Be careful not to lick the bowl.

Mediterranean Baked Tilapia

SmartPoints value: Green plan - 3SP, Blue plan - 1SP, Purple plan - 1SP

Total time: 25 min, Prep time: 10 min, Cooking time: 15 min, Serves: 4

Nutritional value: Calories - 129, Fat - 5g, Protein - 21g

Ingredients

Tilapia fillets - 1 lb (about eight fillets)

Olive oil - 1 tsp

Butter - 1 tbsp

Shallots (finely chopped) - 2 pieces

Garlic (minced) - 3 cloves

Cumin (ground) - 1 1/2 tsp

Paprika (1 1/2 tsp)

Capers (1/4 cup)

Dill (finely chopped, fresh) - 1/4 cup

Lemon juice - from 1 lemon

Pepper and salt to taste

Instructions

1.   Line a rimmed baking sheet with parchment paper or foil over a preheated oven of 375 degrees. Mist with cooking spray and spread fish fillets evenly on the baking sheet.

2.   Combine the paprika, pepper, and salt in a small bowl. Season the fish fillets with the spice mixture on both sides.

3.   Whisk together in a small bowl, the melted butter, olive oil, lemon juice, shallots, and garlic then brush evenly over the fish fillets.

Top with the capers.

4.   Making sure not to overcook, bake in the oven for about 10-15 minutes, then remove from oven and top with fresh dill.

Two-Ingredient Ice Cream

Cupcake Bites

SmartPoints value: Green plan - 2SP, Blue plan - 2SP, Purple plan - 2SP

Total Time: 32 min, Prep time: 5 min, Cooking time: 12 min, Serves: 12

Nutritional value: Calories - 109, Carbs - 10g, Fat - 8g, Protein - 12g

Ingredients

Ice cream bars (WW Dark Chocolate-raspberry) - 6 bar(s) White flour (self-rising) - 10 Tbsp Whipped topping (light) - 4 Tbsp Sprinkles (rainbow) - ½ Tbsp

Instructions

1.   After preheating the oven to 350°F, coat twelve mini muffin holes with cooking spray

2.   Drop the ice cream from the sticks into a large bowl and allow it to melt slightly, then add some white flour and stir until it is well-mixed.

3.   Evenly fill prepared muffin holes with the mixture and bake until a tester inserted in the center of a cupcake comes out without anything sticking to it; about 10-12 minutes.

4.   Allow the cupcakes to cool in the pan for a few minutes before taking them out. Collect the processed muffins from the pan and cool completely.

5.   Put one teaspoon of whipped topping in each cooled cupcake and divide the sprinkles over the top.

Lemon Blueberry Cheesecake Yogurt Bark

SmartPoints value: 1SP

Total time: 1 hr 15 mins, Prep time: 15 mins, Chill time: 1 hr, Serves - 12

Nutritional value: Calories - 124, Carbs - 12.7g, Fat - 0.2g, Protein - 18.2g

Ingredients

Greek yogurt (plain non-fat) - 1 cup

Agave nectar - 1 tablespoon

Lemon zest - 1/2 teaspoon

Lemon juice (fresh-squeezed) - 1/2 teaspoon Blueberries (fresh) - 1 cup

Graham crackers (crushed into crumbs) - 3 squares (gluten-free if you like)

Instructions

1.   Line a 9x5-inch loaf pan with aluminum foil so that the foil hangs over sides of the pan.

2.   Mix the yogurt, lemon zest, agave nectar, and lemon juice in a small mixing bowl, then stir.

3.   Turn in the blueberries gently with three tablespoons crushed graham cracker crumbs just until adequately mixed.

4.   Evenly spread the mixture into the loaf pan you earlier prepared. Get the remaining cracker crumbs and sprinkle over the top.

5.   Use aluminum foil to cover the loaf pan and refrigerate for at least 1 hour; until it is frozen.

6.   Once the mixture is frozen, remove the pan from the freezer and use overhanging foil as handles to lift the bark from the pan.

7.   Put the frozen mixture on a cutting board and slice it into eight squares.

8.   Cut each square diagonally, creating two triangles. (If the frozen dough is too difficult to cut, allow it to sit out at room temperature to soften. Alternatively, you can keep the knife inside hot water before cutting.)

9.   Keep the cut portions in an airtight container inside the freezer until you are ready to serve. Allow the cut triangles to sit on the

table at room temperature to soften slightly before serving if it is too frozen.

Dark Chocolate Avocado Mousse

This chocolate delicacy, loaded with healthy fats, fiber, and antioxidants, is a perfect dessert recipe.

SmartPoints value - 9SP

Total time: 1 hr 10 mins, Prep time: 10 mins, Chill time: 1 hr, Serves: 2

Nutritional value: Calories - 434, Carbs - 53g, Fat - 29g, Protein - 6g

Ingredients

Avocado (very ripe, peeled and seeded) - 1 large

Dark baking chocolate (70% cacao, melted) - 2 ounces

Cocoa powder (unsweetened) - 2 Tbsp

Almond milk (unsweetened) - 1/4 cup

Maple syrup - 2 Tbsp

Pure vanilla extract - 1/4 Tsp

Cinnamon (ground) - A pinch

Salt - A pinch

Instructions

1.   Get a blender and put in avocado, maple syrup, melted chocolate, milk, cocoa powder, vanilla, cinnamon, and salt.

2.   Process the content of the blender until you get a smooth and creamy mixture. To make the mousse thinner, add more milk or less milk for a thicker mousse.

3.   Pour the mixture evenly into two small dessert glasses.

4.   Chill it for at least 1 hour in the refrigerator before serving.

Hearty Chia and Blackberry Pudding

Serving: 2

Prep Time: 45 minutes

Cook Time: Nil

Ingredients:

¼ cup chia seeds

½ cup blackberries, fresh

1 teaspoon liquid sweetener

1 cup coconut almond milk, full fat and unsweetened

1 teaspoon vanilla extract

How To:

1.   Take the vanilla, liquid sweetener and coconut almond milk and add to blender.

2.   Process until thick.

3.   Add in blackberries and process until smooth.

4.   Divide the mixture between cups and chill for 30 minutes.

5.   Serve and enjoy!

Nutrition (Per Serving)

Calories: 437

Fat: 38g

Carbohydrates: 8g

Protein: 8g

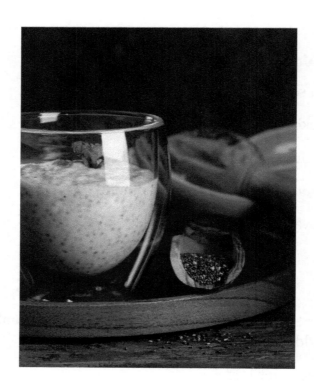

Special Cocoa Brownie Bombs

Serving: 12

Prep Time: 15 minutes

Cooking Time: 25 minutes

Freeze Time: None

Ingredients:

2 tablespoons grass-fed almond butter

1 whole egg

2 teaspoons vanilla extract

¼ teaspoon baking powder

1/3 cup heavy cream

3/4 cup almond butter

¼ cocoa powder

A pinch of sunflower seeds

How To:

1. Break the eggs and whisk until smooth.

2.   Add in all the wet ingredients and mix well.

3.   Make the batter by mixing all the dry ingredients and sifting them into the wet ingredients.

4.   Pour into a greased baking pan.

5.   Bake for 25 minutes at 350 degrees F or until a toothpick inserted in the middle comes out clean.

6.   Let it cool, slice and serve.

Nutrition (Per Serving)

Total Carbs: 1g

Fiber: 0g

Protein: 1g

Fat: 20g

Elegant Mango Compote

Serving: 4

Prep Time: 10 minutes

Cook Time: 10 minutes

Ingredients:

4 cups mango, peeled and cubed

1 cup orange juice

6 tablespoons palm sugar

3 tablespoons lime juice

How To:

1. Add mango, lime juice, orange juice, sugar to your Instant Pot.

2. Lock the lid and cook on LOW pressure for 10 minutes.

3. Release the pressure naturally over 10 minutes.

4. Remove the lid and divide amongst serving bowls.

5. Enjoy!

Nutrition (Per Serving)

Calories: 180

Fat: 2g

Carbohydrates: 12g

Protein: 2g

Lovely Carrot Cake

Prep Time: 3 hours 15 minutes

Cooking Time: Ni

Serving: 6

Ingredients:

For Cashew Frosting

2 tablespoons lemon juice

2 cups cashews, soaked

2 tablespoons coconut oil, melted 1/3 cup maple syrup water

For Cake

1 cup pineapple, dried and chopped

2 carrots, chopped

1 ½ cups coconut flour

1 cup dates, pitted

½ cup dry coconut

½ teaspoon cinnamon

How To:

1.   Add cashews, lemon juice, maple syrup, coconut oil, apple and pulse well.

2.   Transfer to a bowl and keep it on the side.

3.   Add carrots to your processor and pulse a few times.

4.   Add flour, dates, pineapple, coconut, cinnamon and pulse.

5.   Pour half of the mixture into a spring form pan and spread well.

6.   Add 1/3 of the cashew frosting and spread evenly.

7.   Add remaining cake batter and spread the frosting.

8.   Place in your freezer until it is hard.

9.   Cut and serve.

10.   Enjoy!

Nutrition (Per Serving)

Calories: 140

Fat: 4g

Carbohydrates: 8g

Protein: 4g

Grilled Peach with Honey Yogurt Dressing

Prep Time: 10 minutes
Cooking Time: 5 minutes
Serving: 6

Ingredients:

2 large peaches, ripe and halved

2 tablespoons honey

1/8 teaspoon cinnamon

¼ cut vanilla Greek yogurt, fat free

How To:

1.   Prepare your outdoor grill and heat on low heat.
2.   Grill your peaches on indirect heat until they are tender,
it should take about 2-4 minutes each side.
3.   Take a bowl and mix in yogurt and cinnamon.
4.   Drizzle honey mix on top and enjoy!

Nutrition (Per Serving)
Calories: 140
Fat: 4g
Carbohydrates: 8g
Protein: 4g

Hearty Carrot Cookies

Prep Time: 10 minutes

Cooking Time: 15 minutes

Serving: 6

Ingredients:

½ cup packed light brown sugar

½ cup sugar

½ cup oil

½ cup apple sauce

2 whole eggs

1 cup flour

1 teaspoon vanilla

1 teaspoon baking soda

1 cup whole wheat flour

¼ teaspoon salt

½ teaspoon ground nutmeg

1 teaspoon cinnamon, ground

1 ½ cups carrots, grated

1 cup golden raisin

2 cups rolled oats, raw

How To:

1.	Pre-heat your oven to about 350 degrees F.

2.	Take a bowl and mix in applesauce, oil, sugar, vanilla and eggs.

3.	Take another bowl and mix in the dry ingredients.

4.	Blend the dry ingredients into the bowl with wet mixture.

5.	Stir in carrots and raisins to the mix.

6.	Take a greased cookie sheet and drop in the mixture spoon by spoon.

7.	Transfer to oven and bake for 15 minutes until you have a golden-brown texture.

8.	Serve and enjoy!

Nutrition (Per Serving)

Calories: 140

Fat: 4g

Carbohydrates: 8g

Protein: 4g

Milky Pudding

Prep Time: 10 minutes

Cooking Time: 5-10 minutes + chill time

Serving: 6

Ingredients:

3 tablespoons cornstarch

½ teaspoon vanilla

1/3 cup chocolate chips

2 cups non-fat milk

1/8 teaspoon salt

2 tablespoons salt

2 tablespoons sugar

How To:

1.   Take a medium sized bowl and add cocoa powder, cornstarch, salt, sugar and mix well.

2.   Whisk in the milk.

3.   Place over medium heat and keep heating until thick and bubbly.

4.   Remove the mixture from heat and stir in vanilla and chocolate chips.

5.   Keep mixing until the chips are melted and you have a smooth pudding.

6.   Pour into a large sized dish and let it chill.

7.   Serve and enjoy!

Nutrition:

Calories: 140

Fat: 4g

Carbohydrates: 8g

Protein: 4g

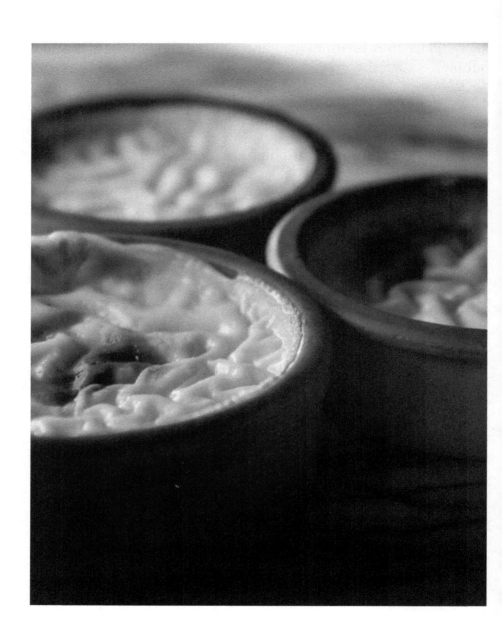

Fresh Honey Strawberries with Yogurt

Prep Time: 10 minutes
Cooking Time: 5-10 minutes + chill time
Serving: 6

Ingredients:

4 tablespoons almond, sliced and toasted
3 cups yogurt, low fat
4 teaspoons honey
1-pint fresh strawberries

How To:

1.   Take your strawberries and wash under water, clean well.
2.   Cut into quarters.
3.   Take your serving dishes and add ¾ cup yogurt into each dish.
4.   Divide strawberries among the dishes.
5.   Top each dish with honey, sliced almonds.
6.   Serve and enjoy!

Nutrition:
Calories: 140
Fat: 4g
Carbohydrates: 8g
Protein: 4g

Spinach Dip

Serving: 2

Prep Time: 4 minutes

Cook Time: 0 minutes

Ingredients:

5 ounces Spinach, raw

1 cup Greek yogurt

1/2 tablespoon onion powder

1/4 teaspoon garlic sunflower seeds

Black pepper to taste

1/4 teaspoon Greek Seasoning

How To:

1.   Add the listed ingredients in a blender.

2.   Emulsify.

3.   Season and serve.

Nutrition (Per Serving)

Calories: 101

Fat: 4g

Carbohydrates: 4g

Protein: 10g

Cauliflower Rice

Serving: 2

Prep Time: 5 minutes

Cook Time: 6 minutes

Ingredients:

1 head grated cauliflower head

1 tablespoon coconut aminos

1 pinch of sunflower seeds

1 pinch of black pepper

1 tablespoon Garlic Powder

1 tablespoon Sesame Oil

How To:

1.   Add cauliflower to a food processor and grate it.

2.   Take a pan and add sesame oil, let it heat up over medium heat.

3.   Add grated cauliflower and pour coconut aminos.

4.   Cook for 4-6 minutes.

5.   Season and enjoy!

Nutrition (Per Serving)

Calories: 329

Fat: 28g

Carbohydrates: 13g

Protein: 10g

Grilled Sprouts and Balsamic Glaze

Serving: 2

Prep Time: 10 minutes

Cook Time: 30 minutes

Ingredients:

½ pound Brussels sprouts, trimmed and halved Fresh cracked black pepper 1 tablespoon olive oil

Sunflower seeds to taste

2 teaspoons balsamic glaze

2 wooden skewers

How To:

1.   Take wooden skewers and place them on a largely sized foil.

2.   Place sprouts on the skewers and drizzle oil, sprinkle sunflower seeds and pepper.

3.   Cover skewers with foil.

4.	Pre-heat your grill to low and place skewers (with foil) in the grill.

5.	Grill for 30 minutes, making sure to turn after every 5-6 minutes.

6.	Once done, uncovered and drizzle balsamic glaze on top.

7.	Enjoy!

Nutrition (Per Serving)

Calories: 440

Fat: 27g

Carbohydrates: 33g

Protein: 26g

Amazing Green Creamy Cabbage

Serving: 4

Prep Time: 10 minutes

Cook Time: 10 minutes

Ingredients:

2 ounces almond butter

1 ½ pounds green cabbage, shredded

1 ¼ cups coconut cream

Sunflower seeds and pepper to taste

8 tablespoons fresh parsley, chopped

How To:

1.   Take a skillet and place it over medium heat, add almond butter and let it melt.

2.   Add cabbage and sauté until brown.

3.   Stir in cream and lower the heat to low.

4.   Let it simmer.

5.   Season with sunflower seeds and pepper.

6. Garnish with parsley and serve.

7. Enjoy!

Nutrition (Per Serving)

Calories: 432

Fat: 42g

Carbohydrates: 8g

Protein: 4g

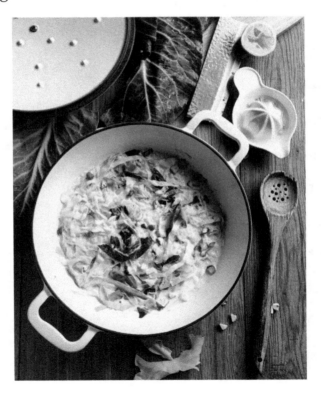

Poached Eggs with Hollandaise and Bacon

SmartPoints value: Green plan – 7SP, Blue plan – 5SP, Purple plan – 5SP

Total Time: 26 min, Prep time: 12 min, Cooking time: 14 min, Serves: 4

Nutritional value: Calories – 677.3, Carbs – 29.2g, Fat – 47.8g, Protein - 31.4g

Ingredients

Plain fat-free yogurt - ¼ cup(s)

Reduced-calorie mayonnaise - ¼ cup(s)

Dijon Mustard - 1 tsp

Uncooked Canadian bacon - 4 slice(s)

Lemon zest - ½ tsp

Egg(s) - 4 item(s), large

Fresh lemon juice - 1 tsp

Fresh tomato(es) - 4 slice(s), thick

Unsalted butter - 2 tsp, softened

Chives - 2 Tbsp, chopped fresh (optional)

English muffin - 2 item(s), multigrain or whole wheat variety, split and toasted

White wine vinegar - 1 Tbsp

Instructions

1. To prepare the sauce, get a small microwavable bowl and whisk yogurt, mayonnaise, mustard, and lemon zest and juice together in the bowl.

2. Set the microwave to High, and allow the mixture to heat up for about 30 seconds. Remove the bowl from the microwave carefully using your mitts.

3. Scoop a tablespoon of butter and stir it in until melted. Cover the bowl to keep your sauce warm.

4. Poach eggs by filling a large, deep skillet with water and allow to boil; add vinegar.

5. Reduce the heat to a bare simmer. Carefully break the eggs into a custard cup, one at a time, and slip into the hot water.

6. Cook the eggs until the whites are firm, but the yolks are still soft. This process should take about 5 minutes.

7. Transfer the eggs, one at a time, with a slotted spoon to a paper towel-lined plate to drain. Cover the plate to keep the eggs warm.

8.   Wipe the skillet dry with a paper towel.

9.   Add four slices of Canadian bacon and cook over medium-high heat until they brown in spots, about 60 seconds per side.

10.   Place one half each of the English muffins on four plates.

11.   Top each with one slice of bacon, one slice of tomato, one poached egg, and about two tablespoons sauce. Speckle with chives, if using.

Note: You can keep the hollandaise sauce warm for up to 40 minutes before serving.

Nut-crusted Mahi-mahi

SmartPoints value: Green plan - 3SP, Blue plan - 2SP, Purple plan - 2SP

Total Time: 20 min, Prep time: 8 min, Cooking time: 12 min, Serves: 4

Nutritional value: Calories - 234.1, Carbs - 13.9g, Fat - 9.8g, Protein - 24.7g

Ingredients

Cooking spray - 2 spray(s)

Egg white(s) (whipped) - 1 large

Macadamia nuts (dry roasted, salted) - 3 Tbsp, chopped

Mahi-mahi fillet(s) (uncooked) - 1 pound(s), no skin

Parsley (fresh) - 2 Tbsp, or cilantro (fresh, minced)

Plain breadcrumbs (dried) - ¼ cup(s), panko (Japanese variety)

Table salt - ¾ tsp (divided)

Instructions

1.   Prepare the oven by preheating to 450°F. Coat a baking pan with cooking spray and place the container in the oven to heat.

2.   Place some nuts, parsley (or cilantro), panko, and 1/4 tsp of salt in a small blender, then blend all together.

3.   Pour the crumbs into a shallow bowl or plate and set the plate aside.

4.   With the fish placed on a plate, rub 1/2 teaspoon of salt all over it.

5.   Dip the fish into the egg white and turn it to coat. After that, dip the fish into the blended nut mixture and turn to coat.

6.   Remove the pan from the oven and place the coated fish on it.

7.   Roast the fish until the center of the fish is no longer translucent; about 10 to 12 minutes. Serve it immediately once it is ready.

Note: If you desire it, you can garnish with salt and pepper, but that could affect the Smart Points value.

Pan-Fried Flounder

SmartPoints value: Green plan - 4SP, Blue plan - 3SP, Purple plan - 3SP

Total Time: 20 min, Prep time: 14 min, Cooking time: 6 min, Serves: 4

Nutritional value: Calories - 441.2, Carbs - 14.8g, Fat - 30.3g, Protein - 8.3g

Ingredients

Black pepper (freshly ground) - ½ tsp (or to taste)

Cornmeal (yellow) - ¼ cup(s)

Dijon mustard - 1 Tbsp

Egg white(s) (whipped) - 1 large

Lemon(s) - ½ medium, cut into four wedges

Olive oil cooking spray - 2 spray(s)

Olive oil - 1 Tbsp

Parmesan cheese (grated) - 2 Tbsp

Thyme (fresh) - 1 Tbsp, or 1 tsp dried thyme

Table salt - ½ tsp (or to taste)

Uncooked flounder fillet(s) - 1 pound(s)

Instructions

1.   Wash the fish with clean water and pat it dry. Place the fish on a plate and sprinkle both sides of fish with mustard, then dip it into the egg white and set aside.

2.   Mix cornmeal, thyme, Parmesan cheese, salt, and pepper in a medium bowl, then dust the fish with cornmeal-mixture. Ensure that to cover both sides.

3.   Get a large oven-proof skillet and coat it with cooking spray, then set it over medium to medium-high heat. Apply heat to the oil until it starts shimmering.

4.   Add the fish to the skillet and cook for 2 to 3 minutes on one side, then flip the fish and cook until it is ready on the other side; about 2 to 3 minutes.

5.   Serve the fish with your lemon wedges.

Blueberry-Almond Oatmeal

SmartPoints value: Green plan - 3SP, Blue plan - 3SP, Purple plan - 1SP

Total time: 10 min, Prep time: 2 min, Cooking time: 5 min, Serves: 1

Nutritional value: Calories - 340, Carbs - 54g Fat - 8g, Protein - 16g

Ingredients

Blueberries (fresh) - ¼ cup(s)

Almond milk (unsweetened) - 2 Tbsp

Slivered almonds - 2 tsp (toasted)

Old-fashioned rolled oats (such as Quaker Oats) - 1 cup

Milk - 1 cup

Water - 1 cup

Kosher salt - 1/8 tsp

Ground cinnamon - 1/2 tsp

Honey - 1 tsp

Instructions

1.   To prepare oatmeal, combine oats, water, milk, salt, and cinnamon in a medium-sized saucepan. Get it to boil on medium-high heat, and reduce heat to low; about 4-5 min.

2.   Simmer it uncovered until it thickens, occasionally stirring. Remove it from the heat and allow to cool slightly.

3.   Stir blueberries and milk into the oatmeal, then sprinkle it with almonds and cinnamon. Add artificial sweetener to taste if you desire.

Toasted Blueberry Muffin with Warm Citrus Compote

SmartPoints value: Green plan - 4SP, Blue plan - 4SP, Purple plan - 4SP

Total Time: 20 min, Prep time: 10 min, Cooking time: 10 min, Serves: 6

Nutritional value: Calories - 231, Carbs - 36.3g Fat - 7.7g, Protein - 5.2g

Ingredients

Brown sugar (Splenda) blend - 1 tsp

Cornstarch - 1 Tbsp

Water - 2 Tbsp

Orange juice (fresh) - ½ cup(s)

Orange sections - 1 cup(s), divided

Vanilla extract - ⅛ teaspoon

Lemon zest - ⅛ teaspoon

Lime zest - ⅛ teaspoon

WW Blueberry muffin - 3 item(s)

Instructions

1.   Prepare the oven by preheating to 350°F.

2.   Whisk cornstarch, brown sugar, and water together in a medium-sized saucepan.

3.   Whip the mixture in orange juice. While whipping constantly, bring the mixture to a boil over medium heat; about 2 minutes. The mixture will thicken rapidly, so make sure to whisk continuously to prevent lumps.

4.   Whisk the thick mixture in half cup of orange segments and continue to simmer over medium-low heat for another 6 to 8 minutes, stirring it regularly. The orange sections should break down, and the sauce should become thick, but it should not stiffen up.

5.   Drop the thick sauce from the heat and stir in vanilla extract, lemon zest, and lime zest. Allow it to cool off for about 10 minutes.

6.   While the sauce is getting cooled, cut each muffin in half and toast them in the oven lightly on both sides.

7.   Serve each person half a muffin topped with two tablespoons of compote. Garnish them with the remaining half cup of orange segments.

Cuban Black Beans and Rice

SmartPoints value: Green plan - 7SP, Blue plan - 4SP, Purple plan - 4SP

Total Time: 35 min, Prep time: 10 min, Cooking time: 25 min, Serves: 6

Nutritional value: Calories - 333.5, Carbs - 54.8g Fat - 5.1g, Protein - 16.1g

Ingredients

Water - 2½ cup(s), divided

Uncooked white rice (long grain-variety) - 1 cup(s)

Olive oil - 2 tsp

Banana pepper(s) - 1 medium

Black beans (canned) - 31 oz, two 15.5 oz cans (undrained)

Cilantro (fresh, chopped, divided) - ⅔ cup(s)

Minced garlic - 1½ Tbsp

Ground cumin - 1 tsp

Uncooked red onion(s) (chopped) - 1¾ cup(s)

Oregano (dried) - 1 tsp

Table salt - 1 tsp (or to taste)

Red wine vinegar - 1 Tbsp

Lime(s) (fresh) - 1 medium, cut into six wedges

Instructions

1.   Bring two cups of water to a boil in a small saucepan and add the rice, then cook as package directs.

2.   Heat some oil in a large nonstick skillet over medium-high heat.

3.   Add a cup of chopped onions and all of the pepper, then cook, occasionally stirring, until it is tender; about 7 minutes.

4.   Toss in garlic, cumin, and oregano, then cook, stirring until fragrant; about 30 seconds.

5.   Stir in the beans and their liquid, the remaining half cup of water and salt, then bring to a simmer.

6.   Reduce the heat to low and simmer for the flavors to blend in about 5 minutes.

7.   Remove the dish from heat, then stir in vinegar and 1/3 cup of cilantro.

8.   To serve, use a spoon to put beans over rice and sprinkle it with 1/4 cup of the remaining onion and 1/3 cup of the remaining cilantro, then squeeze fresh lime juice over the top.

Note: If you desire, sprinkle the dish with salt before serving.

Spaghetti Squash with Fresh Tomato-Basil Sauce

SmartPoints value: Green plan - 2SP, Blue plan - 2SP, Purple plan - 2SP

Total time: 30 min, Prep time: 15 min, Cooking time: 15 min, Serves: 4

Nutritional value: Calories - 216.2, Carbs - 14.2g Fat - 17.2g, Protein - 5.0g

Enjoy this recipe with its taste of summer. Ensure to cook it with very ripe tomatoes and fresh basil to get the best flavour.

Ingredients

Tomato(es) (fresh) - 2¼ pound(s)

Olive oil (extra virgin) - 2 Tbsp

Minced garlic - 1¼ tsp, finely minced

Basil (fresh, sliced) - ½ cup(s)

Kosher salt - ½ tsp (or to taste)

Black pepper (freshly ground) - ¼ tsp (or to taste)

Spaghetti squash (uncooked) - 2½ pound(s)

Instructions

1.   Toss tomatoes, oil, garlic, basil, salt and pepper together in a large bowl and let it stand, occasionally tossing, until the tomatoes release their juices and the mixture is quite juicy; about 10 to 15 minutes.

2.   Cut the spaghetti squash in half and scoop out the seeds, then place the squash in a covered microwave-safe container.

3.   Cook the spaghetti squash on high power until strands of squash separate when you scrape the flesh with a fork; about 15 minutes. Alternatively, you can also roast the squash for about 20 minutes in the oven.

4.   Scrape the spaghetti squash from the peel with a fork to form strands and add it to the bowl with tomatoes and toss to coat.

Notes: It would be delicious to add chunks of fresh mozzarella or freshly grated Parmesan cheese to this meal. However, it might affect the Smart Points value.

Sweet Corn Soup

Nutritional Facts

servings per container	5
Prep Total	**10 min**
Serving Size 2/3 cup (27g)	
Amount per serving **Calories**	**200**
	% Daily Value
Total Fat 8g	**1%**
Saturated Fat 1g	2%
Trans Fat 0g	2%
Cholesterol	**2%**
Sodium 240mg	**7%**
Total Carbohydrate 12g	**2%**
Dietary Fiber 4g	14%
Total Sugar 12g	01.21%
Protein 3g	
Vitamin C 2mcg	2%
Calcium 20mg	1%
Iron 7mg	2%
Potassium 25mg	6%

Ingredients

6 ears of corn

1 tablespoon of corn oil

1 small onion

1/2 cup grated celery root

7 cups water or vegetable stock

Add salt to taste

Instructions:

1. Shuck the corn & slice off the kernels

2. In a large soup pot put in the oil, onion, celery root, and one cup of water

3. Let that mixture stew under low heat until the onion is soft

4. Include the corn, salt & remaining water and bring it to a boil

5. Cool briefly & then puree in a blender, then wait for it to cool before putting it through a food mill.

6. Reheat & add salt with pepper to taste nice.

Mexican Avocado Salad

Nutritional Facts

servings per container	6
Prep Total	**10 min**
Serving Size 2/3 cup (70g)	
Amount per serving **Calories**	**120**
	% Daily Value
Total Fat 8g	**10%**
Saturated Fat 1g	8%
Trans Fat 0g	21
Cholesterol	**22%**
Sodium 16mg	**7%**
Total Carbohydrate 7g	**13%**
Dietary Fiber 4g	14%
Total Sugar 1g	-
Protein 2g	
Vitamin C 1mcg	1%
Calcium 260mg	20%
Iron 2mg	25%
Potassium 235mg	6%

Ingredients

24 cherry tomatoes, quartered

2 tablespoon extra-virgin olive oil

4 teaspoons red wine vinegar

2 teaspoon salt

¼ teaspoon freshly ground black pepper

Gently chopped ½ medium yellow or white onion

1 jalapeño, seeded & finely chopped

2 tablespoons chopped fresh cilantro

¼ medium head iceberg lettuce, cut into ½-inch ribbons
Chopped 2 ripe Hass avocados, seeded, peeled

Instructions:

1.   Add tomatoes, oil, vinegar, salt, & pepper in a neat medium bowl. Add onion, jalapeño & cilantro; toss well

2.   Put lettuce on a platter & top with avocado

3.   Spoon tomato mixture on top and serve.

Crazy Delicious Raw Pad Thai

Nutritional Facts

servings per container	3
Prep Total	**10 min**
Serving Size 2/3 cup (77g)	
Amount per serving **Calories**	**210**
	% Daily Value
Total Fat 3g	**10%**
Saturated Fat 2g	8%
Trans Fat 7g	-
Cholesterol	**0%**
Sodium 120mg	7%
Total Carbohydrate 77g	**10%**
Dietary Fiber 4g	14%
Total Sugar 12g	-
Protein 3g	
Vitamin C 1mcg	20%
Calcium 260mg	20%
Iron 2mg	41%
Potassium 235mg	1%

Ingredients

2 large zucchini

Thinly sliced ¼ red cabbage

Chopped ¼ cup fresh mint leaves

Sliced 1 spring onion

peeled and sliced ½ avocado

10 raw almonds

4 tablespoonful sesame seeds Dressing

¼ cup peanut butter

2 tablespoonful tahini

2 lemon, juiced

2 tablespoonful tamari / salt-reduced soy sauce and add ½ chopped green chili

Instructions:

1.   Collect dressing ingredients in a container

2.   Pop the top on and shake truly well to join. I like mine pleasant and smooth however you can include a dash of sifted water on the off chance that it looks excessively thick.

3.   Using a mandoline or vegetable peeler, expel one external portion of skin from every zucchini and dispose of.

4.   Combine zucchini strips, cabbage & dressing in a vast blending bowl and blend well

5.   Divide zucchini blend between two plates or bowls

6.   Top with residual fixings and appreciate!

Kale and Wild Rice Stir Fly

Nutritional Facts

servings per container	3
Prep Total	**10 min**
Serving Size 2/3 cup (80g)	
Amount per serving **Calories**	**220**
	% Daily Value
Total Fat 5g	**22%**
Saturated Fat 1g	8%
Trans Fat 0g	-
Cholesterol	**0%**
Sodium 200mg	**7%**

Ingredients

1 tablespoonful extra virgin olive oil

Diced ¼ onion

3 carrots, cut into ½ inch slices

2 cups assorted mushrooms

2 bunch kale, chopped into bite-sized pieces

2 tablespoonful lemon juice

2 tablespoonful chili flakes, more if desired

1 tablespoon Braggs Liquid Aminos

2 cup wild rice, cooked

Instructions:

1.   In a large sauté pan, heat oil over on heater. Include onion & cook until translucent, for 35 to 10 minutes.

2.   Include carrots & sauté for another 2 minutes. Include mushrooms & cook for 4 minutes. Include kale, lemon juice, chili flakes & Braggs. Cook until kale is slightly wilted.

3.   Serve over wild rice and enjoy your Lunch!

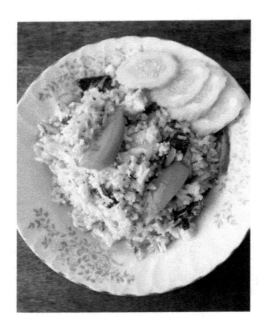

Creamy Avocado Pasta

servings per container	7
Prep Total	**10 min**
Serving Size 2/3 cup (25g)	
Amount per serving **Calories**	19
	% Daily Value
Total Fat 8g	**300%**
Saturated Fat 1g	40%
Trans Fat 0g	20%
Cholesterol	**6%**
Sodium 210mg	**3%**
Total Carbohydrate 22g	**400%**
Dietary Fiber 4g	1%
Total Sugar 12g	02.20%
Protein 3g	
Vitamin C 2mcg	20%
Calcium 10mg	6%
Iron 4mg	7%
Potassium 25mg	6%

Ingredients

340 g / 12 oz spaghetti

2 ripe avocados, halved, seeded & neatly peeled 1/2 cup fresh basil leaves

3 cloves garlic

1/3 cup olive oil

2-3 teaspoon freshly squeezed lemon juice

Add sea salt & black pepper, to taste

1.5 cups cherry tomatoes, halved

Instructions:

1.   In a large pot of boiling salted water, cook pasta according to the package. When al dente, drain and set aside.

2.   To make the avocado sauce, combine avocados, basil, garlic, oil, and lemon juice in food processor. Blend on high until smooth. Season with salt and pepper to taste.

3.   In a large bowl, combine pasta, avocado sauce, and cherry tomatoes until evenly coated.

4.   To serve, top with additional cherry tomatoes, fresh basil, or lemon zest.

5.   Best when fresh. Avocado will oxidize over time so store leftovers in a covered container in refrigerator up to one day.

Zucchini Pasta with Pesto Sauce

Nutritional Facts

servings per container	5
Prep Total	**10 min**
Serving Size 2/3 cup (20g)	
Amount per serving **Calories**	**100**
	% Daily Value
Total Fat 8g	12%
Saturated Fat 1g	2%
Trans Fat 0g	20%
Cholesterol	**2%**
Sodium 10mg	7%
Total Carbohydrate 7g	**2%**
Dietary Fiber 2g	14%
Total Sugar 1g	01.20%
Protein 3g	
Vitamin C 2mcg	10%
Calcium 240mg	1%
Iron 2mg	2%
Potassium 25mg	6%

Ingredients

1 to 2 medium zucchini (make noodles with a mandoline or Spiralizer)

1/2 teaspoon of salt

For Pesto

soaked 1/4 cup cashews

soaked 1/4 cup pine nuts

1/2 cup spinach

1/2 cup peas you can make it fresh or frozen one

1/4 cup broccoli

1/4 cup basil leaves

1/2 avocado

1 or 2 tablespoons original olive oil

2 tablespoons nutritional yeast

1/2 teaspoon salt

Pinch black pepper

Instructions:

1.   Place zucchini noodles in a strainer over a clean bowl

2.   Include 1/2 teaspoon of salt & let it set while preparing the pesto sauce

3.   Mix all the ingredients for the pesto sauce

4.   Extract excess water from zucchini noodles & place them in a clean bowl

5.   Pour the sauce on top & garnish with some basil leaves & pine nut

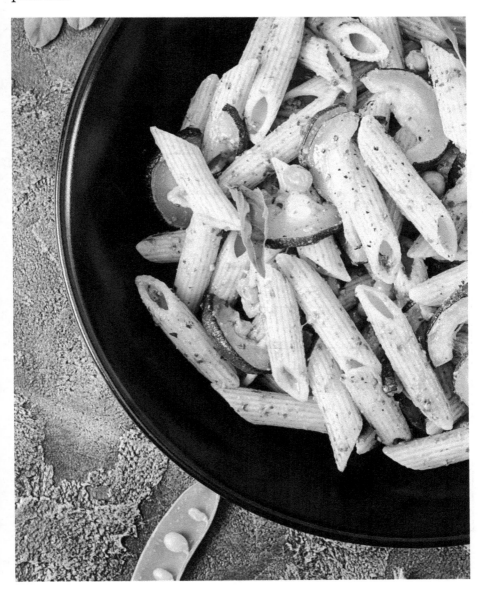

Balsamic BBQ Seitan and Tempeh Ribs

Nutritional Facts

servings per container	4
Prep Total	**10 min**
Serving Size 2/3 cup (56g)	
Amount per serving **Calories**	**100**
	% Daily Value
Total Fat 7g	**1%**
Saturated Fat 1g	2%
Trans Fat 0g	20%
Cholesterol	**2%**
Sodium 160mg	7%
Total Carbohydrate 37g	**2%**
Dietary Fiber 2g	1%
Total Sugar 2g	01.20%
Protein 14g	
Vitamin C 1mcg	10%
Calcium 450mg	1%
Iron 2mg	2%
Potassium 35mg	7%

Ingredients

For the spice rub

Minced ¼ cup fresh parsley

Instructions:

1.   In a clean bowl, join the ingredients for the spice rub. Blend well & put aside.

2.   In a small saucepan over medium heat, combine the apple juice vinegar, balsamic vinegar, maple syrup, ketchup, red onion, garlic, and chile. Mix & let stew, revealed, for around 60 minutes. Increase the level of the heat to medium-high & cook for 15 additional minutes until the sauce thickens. Mix it frequently. In the event that it appears to be excessively thick, include some water.

3.   Preheat the oven to 350 degrees. In a clean bowl, join the dry ingredients for the seitan & blend well. In a clean bowl, add the wet ingredients. Add the wet ingredients to the dry & blend until simply consolidated. Manipulate the dough gently until everything is combined & the dough feels elastic.

4.   Grease or shower a preparing dish. Include the dough to the baking dish, smoothing it & stretching it to fit the dish. Cut the dough into 7 to 9 strips & afterward down the middle to make 16 thick ribs.

5.   Top the dough with the flavor rub & back rub it in a bit. Heat the seitan for 40 minutes to an hour or until the seitan has a strong surface to it. Remove the dish from the heater. Recut the strips & cautiously remove them from the baking dish.

6.   Increase the oven temperature to about 400 degrees. Slather the ribs with BBQ sauce & lay them on a baking sheet.

Set the ribs back in the heater for pretty much 12 minutes so the sauce can get a bit roasted.

Then again, you can cook the sauce-covered ribs on a grill or in a grill pan.

Green Bean Casserole

Nutritional Facts

Serving per container	2
Prep Total	**10 min**
Serving Size 2/3 cup (5g)	
Amount per serving **Calories**	**100**
	% Daily Value
Total Fat 10g	**12%**
Saturated Fat 2g	2%
Trans Fat 4g	20%
Cholesterol	**2%**
Sodium 70mg	7%
Total Carbohydrate 18g	**2%**
Dietary Fiber 9g	10%
Total Sugar 16g	01.20%
Protein 2g	
Vitamin C 9mcg	10%
Calcium 720mg	1%
Iron 6mg	2%
Potassium 150mg	6%

Ingredients

Diced 1 large onion

3 tablespoons of original olive oil

¼ cup flour

2 cups of water

1 tablespoon of salt

½ tablespoons of garlic powder

1 or 2 bags frozen green beans (10 ounces each)

1 fried onion

Instructions:

1.   Preheat oven to 350 degrees.

2.   Heat original olive oil in a shallow pan. Include onion & stir occasionally while the onions soften and turn translucent. This takes about 15 to 20 minutes, don't rush it because it gives so much flavor! Once onion is well cooked, include flour & stir well to cook flour. It will be a dry mixture. Include salt & garlic powder. Add some water. Let simmer for about 1 – 2 minutes & allow mixture to thicken. Immediately remove from heat

3.   Pour green beans into a square baking dish & add 2/3 can of onions. Include all of the gravy & stir well to together

4.   Place in oven & cook for 25 to 30 minutes, gravy mixture will be bubbly. Top with remaining fried onions & cook for 4 to 12 minutes more. Serve immediately and enjoy your dinner.

Socca Pizza [Vegan]

Nutritional Facts

servings per container	2
Prep Total	**10 min**
Serving Size 2/3 cup (78g)	
Amount per serving **Calories**	**120**
	% Daily Value
Total Fat 10g	**20%**
Saturated Fat 5g	7%
Trans Fat 6g	27%
Cholesterol	**5%**
Sodium 10mg	**10%**
Total Carbohydrate 4g	**20%**
Dietary Fiber 9g	15%
Total Sugar 12g	01.70%
Protein 6g	
Vitamin C 7mcg	10%
Calcium 290mg	20%
Iron 4mg	2%
Potassium 240mg	7%

Ingredients

Socca Base

1 cup chickpea (garbanzo bean) flour – I used bob's Red Mill Garbanzo Fava Flour

1 or 2 cups of cold, filtered water

1 to 2 tablespoons minced garlic

½ tablespoon of sea salt

2 tablespoons coconut oil (for greasing)

Toppings

Add Tomato-paste

Add Dried Italian herbs (oregano, basil, thyme, rosemary, etc.)

Add Mushrooms

Add Red onion

Add Capsicum/bell pepper

Add Sun-dried tomatoes

Add Kalamata olives

Add Vegan Cheese & Chopped Fresh basil leaves

Instructions:

1.   Pre-heat oven to 350F

2.   In a clean mixing bowl, whisk together garbanzo bean flour & water until there are no lumps remaining. Stir together in garlic 7 sea salt. Allow resting for about 12 minutes to thicken.

3.   Grease 2 - 4 small, shallow dishes/tins with original coconut oil

4.	Pour mixture into a clean dish & bake for about 20 - 15 minutes or until golden brown.

5.	Remove dishes from oven, top with your favorite toppings & vegan cheese (optional) & return to the oven for another 7 - 10 minutes or so.

6.	Remove dishes from oven & allow to sit for a about 2 – 5 minutes before removing pizzas from the dishes. Enjoy your dinner!

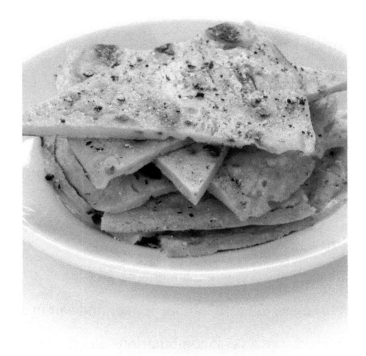

Easy Egg Salad

SmartPoints value: Green plan - 2SP, Blue plan - 2SP, Purple plan - 2SP

Total time: 5 min, Prep time: 5 min, Serves: 2

Nutritional value: Calories - 229, Carbs - 3g, Fat - 17g, Protein - 12g

Ingredients

Hard-boiled eggs - 4 pieces

Olive oil - 1 tbsp

Onions (diced) - 1/3 cup

Paprika - ½ tsp

Pepper and salt to taste

Instructions

1.   Grate the peeled egg using a cheese grater

2.   Mix the eggs, olive oil, onion, pepper and salt in a bowl

3.   Feel free to try several combinations and find your favorite. You could try toppings like tomatoes, dill, parsley, chives, relish, pickles, olives, bell peppers, or avocados.

Summer Green Bean Salad

SmartPoints value: Green plan - 1SP, Blue plan - 1SP, Purple plan - 1SP

Total time: 18 min, Prep time: 15 min, Cooking time: 3 min, Serves:

Nutritional value: Calories - 69, Carbs – 9.1g, Fat – 3.7g, Protein - 2g

Ingredients

Green beans (fresh, cut into pieces) - (1 lb)

Red onion (thinly sliced) - 1/2

Cherry tomatoes (halved) - 1 1/2 cups

Basil (finely chopped, fresh) - 1/2 cup

Garlic (minced) - 2 cloves

Olive oil - 1 1/2 tbsp

Lemon juice - 1 cup

Pepper and salt to taste

Instructions

1.   Boil a pot of water and blanch the green beans in the water for about 3 minutes. Drain the beans and transfer to an ice bath for about 2-3 minutes, then place the dried green beans in a large bowl.

2.   Put the remaining ingredients and toss thoroughly.

3.   Enjoy!

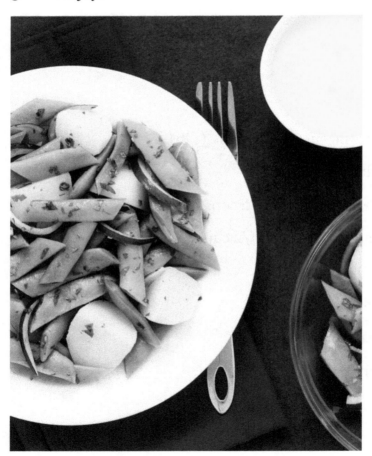

Chopped Greek Salad with Creamy Yogurt Dressing

SmartPoints value: Green plan - 4SP, Blue plan - 4SP, Purple plan - 4SP

Total Time: 20 min, Prep time: 2 min, Cooking time: 18 min, Serves: 6

Nutritional value: Calories - 29.0, Carbs - 0.5g Fat - 2.7g, Protein - 0.8g

Ingredients

Black pepper (freshly ground) - ¼ tsp (or to taste)

Low-fat yogurt (plain) - ¾ cup(s), (not Greek)

Crumbled feta cheese - ½ cup(s)

Dill (fresh, chopped) - 1 Tbsp

Water - 3 Tbsp

Olive oil (extra virgin) - 2 Tbsp

Lemon zest - 1 tsp

Lemon juice (fresh) - 1 Tbsp, (or to taste)

Garlic cloves (very finely minced) - 1 small clove(s)

Oregano (dried) - 1 tsp

Table salt - ½ tsp (or to taste)

Cucumber(s) (English variety, diced) - 1 medium

Yellow pepper(s) (diced) - 2 medium

Grape tomatoes - 2 cup(s), halved

Mint leaves (fresh) - ¾ cup(s), leaves, torn

Uncooked red onion(s) - ⅓ cup(s), chopped

Olive(s) (pitted, sliced) - 12 medium, Kalamata

Instructions

1.	Cut the tomatoes in half, and dice the cucumber, peppers, and onion. Set it aside.

2.	Whip yogurt, oil, water, lemon zest, and juice together in a clean small bowl, then add garlic, dill, oregano, salt, and pepper.

3.	Combine the remaining ingredients inside a large bowl and toss them together. Add the mixture to the dressing, then toss to coat.

Roasted Beet and Wheat Berry

Salad

SmartPoints value: Green plan: 6SP, Blue plan: 6SP, Purple plan: 3SP Total Time: 60 min, Prep time: 20 min, Cooking time: 40 min, Serves: 6 Nutritional value: Calories - 141.4, Carbs - 22.8g Fat - 5.0g, Protein - 6.4g

Ingredients

Cooking spray - 3 spray(s)

Beets (uncooked) - 2 pound(s), red or golden (scrubbed)

Kosher salt - 2½ tsp, divided

Wheat berries (uncooked) - 1 cup(s)

Orange juice (unsweetened) - 2 Tbsp

Orange marmalade - 1 Tbsp

Olive oil (extra-virgin) - 1 Tbsp

Apple cider vinegar - 1 Tbsp

Scallion(s)(uncooked) - ½ cup(s), sliced (white and light green parts), or to taste

Parsley (fresh) - ⅓ cup(s), flat-leaf, chopped, or to taste

Goat cheese (semisoft) - ⅓ cup(s), crumbled

Table salt - ¼ tsp (or to taste)

Black pepper - ¼ tsp (or to taste)

Instructions

1.   Prepare the oven by heating to 400°F. Coat a clean baking pan with cooking spray.

2.   Place beets on the prepared baking pan and lightly coat with cooking spray. Sprinkle the beets with a half teaspoon of salt and tightly cover with foil, then roast until tender; about 40 min.

3.   Remove the pan from the oven and allow beets to cool slightly,

then gently remove the skin with a knife.

4.   Dice the beets or cut into thick matchsticks and set aside.

5.   Cover wheatberries with two inches of water in a small saucepan and stir in one teaspoon of salt, then bring it to a boil.

6.   Reduce the heat to low, cover it, and simmer until the wheat berries are tender; about 50 - 60 minutes. Drain the saucepan and set aside.

7.   To make a vinaigrette, mix orange juice, marmalade, oil, vinegar and remaining teaspoon salt in a small bowl, while the beets and wheatberries cook.

8.   Use a clean spoon to put the wheat berries into a serving bowl and gently toss them with the beets, vinaigrette, scallions and parsley, then season to taste with salt and pepper.

9.   Garnish the dish with goat cheese and serve.

Italian Pasta Salad with Tomatoes and Artichoke Hearts

SmartPoints value: Green plan - 5SP, Blue plan - 5SP, Purple plan - 5SP

Total Time: 28 min, Prep time: 18 min, Cooking time: 10 min, Serves: 6

Nutritional value: Calories - 296.2, Carbs - 47.3g Fat - 8.2g, Protein - 8.7g

Ingredients

Tomato(es) (fresh) - 1 pound(s), ripe beefsteak or Campari, chopped (3 cups)

Bell pepper(s) (uncooked) - 2 item(s), small, yellow and orange, diced (1 ½ cups)

Artichoke hearts without oil (canned) - 14 oz, drained, roughly chopped

Basil (torn or coarsely chopped) - 1 cup(s)

Red wine vinegar - 2 Tbsp

Olive oil (extra virgin) - 2 Tbsp

Table salt - ½ tsp, with extra for cooking pasta

Black pepper - ½ tsp, freshly ground

Garlic powder - ¼ tsp, or more to taste

Pasta (uncooked) - 6 oz, cellentani recommended (2 cups)
Parmesan cheese (shredded) - ⅓ cup(s), or shaved, divided

Instructions

1.   Combine artichoke hearts, basil, tomatoes, peppers, vinegar, oil, salt, pepper, and garlic powder in a large bowl, then toss to coat. Allow the pasta to stand while cooking, occasionally tossing.

2.   Boil a pot of well-salted water and cook the pasta according to package directions. Drain and rinse it with cold water, then drain again.

3.   Add the pasta to the bowl with tomato mixture and toss to coat. Add all but two Tbsp Parmesan and toss again.

4.   Serve the pasta salad with the remaining cheese sprinkled over to the top.

Tofu-veggie Kebabs with Peanut-sriracha Sauce

SmartPoints value: Green plan: 7SP, Blue plan - 3SP, Purple plan - 3SP

Total Time: 41 min, Prep time: 35 min, Cooking time: 6 min, Serves: 4

Nutritional value: Calories - 144.7, Carbs - 9.5g Fat - 8.9g, Protein - 8.8g

Ingredients

Broccoli (uncooked) - 10 oz, florets (about 4 cups)

Cooking spray - 4 spray(s)

Firm tofu (rinsed and drained) - 28 oz

Table salt - ½ tsp

Radish(es) (fresh, trimmed and halved) - 8 medium

Lime juice (fresh) - 1½ Tbsp

Peanut butter (powdered) - 6 Tbsp

Water - 4½ Tbsp

Ketchup - 3 Tbsp

White miso - 3 Tbsp, (low-sodium)

Soy sauce (low-sodium) - 1½ Tbsp

Sriracha hot sauce - 1½ tsp

Sesame oil (toasted) - 1½ tsp

Sesame seeds (unsalted toasted) - 1 Tbsp

Instructions

1.   Soak up to eight 10-inches bamboo skewers in a shallow dish containing water for at least 20 minutes (or use metal skewers).

2.   Put water in a large saucepan and bring it to a boil over high heat. Add salt and radishes to the pan and cook for 5 minutes.

3.   Add broccoli and cook for 1 minute more. Drain a colander into the saucepan and its content, then Dash the vegetables under cold water until it is cool to the touch. Drain it properly; Pat it dry with paper towels.

4.   Dry out the tofu blocks with paper towels and cut each block into 12 even cubes.

5.   To prepare the sauce, stir the water and powdered peanut butter together in a medium bowl to form a smooth, loose paste.

6.   Add lime juice, ketchup, miso, Sriracha, soy sauce, and oil, then stir to mix.

7.   To prepare kebabs, thread two broccoli florets, two radish

halves, and three tofu cubes on each skewer.

8.   Apply medium-high heat to a grill. Brush the kebabs with sauce on one side and lightly coat with cooking spray off the heat.

9.   Place the kebabs on the grill, sauce side down and cook for 2-3 minutes.

10.   Brush the other side with the sauce, flip it and cook for another 2-3 minutes.

11.   Remove the kebabs from the grill and brush them with extra sauce, then sprinkle them with sesame seeds before serving.

Crockpot Beef Stew

SmartPoints value: Green plan - 6SP, Blue plan - 6SP, Purple plan - 6SP

SmartPoints value: Green plan - 6SP, Blue plan - 6SP, Purple plan - 6SP

Total Time: 1hr 15min, Prep time: 15 min, Cooking time: 1hr, Serves: 8

Nutritional value: Calories – 343, Carbs – 23.5g, Fat – 17.3g, Protein – 22.2g

Ingredients

Beef chuck roast - 2 lb

Russet potatoes (2-in diameter) - 4 medium

Carrots - 4 medium

Onion - 1 large

Garlic - 4 cloves

Onion soup mix - 1 packet

Fat-free beef broth - 8 cups

Celery stalks (chopped) - 4 medium

Add salt and pepper (to taste)

Instructions

1.   Chop the roast into pieces (1 inch)

2.   Cut peeled potatoes into slices (1/2 inch)

3.   Cut peeled carrots into equal chunks (1/2 inch)

4.   Cut onion into large pieces

5.   Mix the beef, celery, carrots, potatoes, onion, garlic, onion soup mix and beef broth inside the crockpot

6.   Add seasoning to taste (salt and pepper)

7.   Cook till it's ready

8.   This meal is easy to prepare. All you need to do is give it a try and enjoy it.

Chicken, Lentil, and Spinach Soup

SmartPoints value: Green plan - 1SP, Blue plan - 1SP, Purple plan - 1SP

Total Time: 1hr 10min, Prep time: 10 min, Cooking time: 1hr, Serves: 6

Nutritional value: Calories – 254, Carbs – 27g, Fat – 4.8g, Protein – 26g

Ingredients

Chicken breast - 1 lb

French dried (green lentils) - 1 cup

Fresh spinach - One 6 oz package

Finely chopped onion (1 piece)

Carrots (chopped) - 2 pieces

Stalk of celery (chopped) - 2 pieces

Garlic (chopped) - 6 cloves

Olive oil (1 tbsp)

Tomato paste - 2 tbsp

Paprika - 1 tsp

Chicken broth or water - 6 cups (fat-free)

Fresh lemon juice – Half a cup

Add salt and pepper to taste

Instructions

1.   Use medium heat to heat olive oil in a large pot or Dutch oven

2.   Put carrots, celery, onions, and garlic and cook till about minutes when vegetables begin to soften

3.   Coat the vegetables with the tomato paste and cover till about 2-3 minutes when the paste begins to darken.

4.   Stir lentils, paprika, salt, and pepper in the broth or water and bring to a boil and add in the chicken, then cook for about 5 minutes.

5.   Cover and cook for about 35 – 45 minutes on medium-low heat until chicken cooks and lentil are tender but not mushy. Make sure the soup is not bubbling or boiling much as you stir periodically.

6.   Shred the chicken breasts using two forks. Stir in spinach and lemon juice and cook for about 2 minutes until the spinach wilts. Turn off the heat and add additional salt and pepper to taste.

7.   To enjoy the chicken stew and leave it in mind as your best, do not overcook the lentils. Keep an eye on it and make sure they are tender but firm.

Roasted Tomato Basil Soup

SmartPoints value: Green plan - 4SP, Blue plan - 4SP, Purple plan - 4SP

Total Time: 1hr 20min, Prep time: 10 min, Cooking time: 1hr 10mins

Serves: 4

Nutritional value: Calories – 238, Carbs – 26.1g, Fat – 3g, Protein – 5g

Most tomato soups are creamy but unfortunately has lots of fat, but this roasted tomato basil soup makes the difference. You might just say goodbye to canned tomato soup after enjoying the fresh flavors of roasted tomato basil soup.

Ingredients

Plum tomatoes (halved) - 2 lbs

Plum tomatoes in their juice - One 14 oz can

Olive oil - 1 tbsp

Onion (diced) - 1 large

Minced garlic (4 cloves)

Butter (2 tbsp)

Red pepper flakes (crushed) - 1/8 tsp

Vegetable stock - 3 cups

Basil (fresh) - 2 cups

Oregano (dried) - 1 tsp

Salt and pepper as desired

Instructions

1. Line a rimmed baking sheet with parchment paper on a 400-degree preheated oven. Before placing them on the baking sheet, toss the tomatoes and garlic cloves with olive oil. Then roast for about 35-45 minutes or until tomatoes are charred.

2. Using medium heat, heat the butter in a stockpot or Dutch, then add onions and red pepper flakes. Sauté until the onion starts to brown.

3. In the canned tomato, stir the basil, oregano, and stock or water. Then, add in the oven-roasted tomatoes and garlic, including any juices on the baking sheet. Boil and simmer uncovered for about 25-30, then stir regularly.

4. Until you reach the desired consistency, process the soup using an immersion blender.

5. Add salt and pepper to taste.

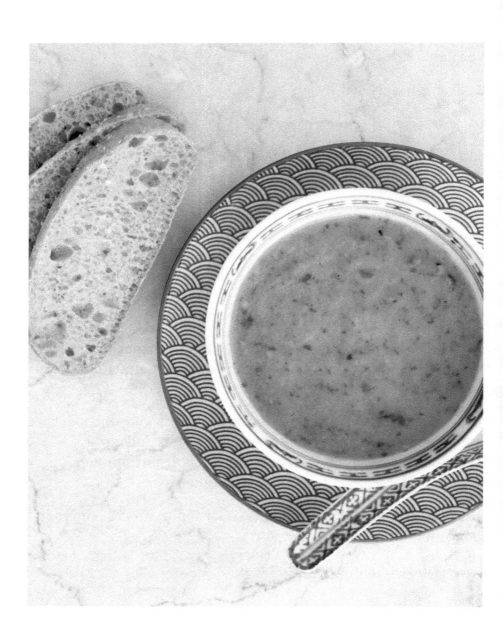